J H ROSCOW

FOREST THERAPY

Thank you to my dearest family and friends, who believed in me. I am eternally grateful for all your help and support.

"In the heart of the forest I find peace and
strength"

- J H Roscow

Contents

Acknowledgement

As we turn the pages of this book, I want to pause and express my deepest gratitude to you, dear reader. Writing this book has been a journey filled with challenges and discoveries that I could not have embarked on without your support. Thank you for dedicating your time and diving into the pages of my story. It means the world to me.

In addition, as a Member of the Woodland Trust. I am beyond grateful for this, and it brings me great passion to be a part of such an incredible team of great volunteers.

(Registered Office) Woodland Trust
Kempton Way, Grantham, Lincolnshire NG31 6LL
General enquiries to: 0330 333 3300
Email: enquiries@woodlandtrust.org.uk

Thank you once again for reading. May you carry a piece of this story with you, as I will carry the memory of this shared journey. If you found this book helpful, I'd be very appreciative if you left a favorable review for the book on Amazon. Until our paths cross again,

J H Roscow

Introduction

Welcome to my little book of Forest Therapy Embracing Nature's Serenity for Health and Well-being. I'm extremely excited to be writing this book! For one it gives me the opportunity to share with you the exceptional benefits of this remarkable experience. And for those who never tried, I urge you to go ahead and see how exhilarating it makes you feel.

I grew up in a small town in Lancashire, there were five of us including mum & dad. I would reminisce about the wonderful memories of our walks, be it home or on holiday, through the wood's valley's nearby rivers, canals, hills and mountains. We've had many magical moments, these wonderful memories have always been a big part of our lives, they have brought so much joy and happiness over the years.

When my husband and I had our own family, we walked in the woods in Keldy North Yorkshire on holiday staying in log cabins deep in the woods. We would pack a van with all the supplies we needed for the four of us, not to mention our bikes, Keldy had outstanding cycle routes. Pick the lads up from school and off we went. I'd make a lovely meat and potato pie for when we arrived at the cabin. Happy Days!

The other reason I'm so excited to write this book is the joy of wanting to share something you love with others. Through this book, I invite readers to experience the beauty and serenity of your environment, hoping to evoke similar feelings of wonder and happiness.

A brief background about myself .... I've experienced quite a lot of traveling over the years, one place in particular I love is the Isle of Man which is a small Island located in the Irish Sea between Britain and Ireland. My adventures in the forest bathing took place in early spring of 2022. It was during the serene, blossoming early spring 2022 that my first adventures of forest bathing unfolded, amidst the tranquil and rejuvenating woodlands of the Isle of Man.

My son and I walked for a while through the woods of Archallagan Forest in the Isle of Man, barefoot feeling the ground under our feet. Oh the feeling of moss is like a lush, natural carpet, cool and slightly damp. It compresses softly under your weight. The moss's velvety surface caresses your skin, a sensation that's both refreshing and soothing.

The tree bark can range from slightly offering a distinct experience. Depending on the type of tree, it can range from slightly rough to deeply grooved. As your feet make contact with the bark, you feel its rugged texture beneath your soles. The bark's firmness provides a stable platform, its irregularities stimulate the pressure points on your feet, invigorating your senses. Walking over bark is a tactile exploration, where each step is a conversation with the tree itself, telling stories of growth, survival, and resilience.

Sharing this experience with my son can strengthen our emotional bond. It's a chance for uninterrupted conversation, sharing thoughts and feelings, or simply enjoying each other's company in silence. These moments can become cherished memories for both of us.

In a world increasingly dominated by screens and indoor activities, walking barefoot in the woods is a great way to encourage physical activity. It helps build a healthy lifestyle habit, emphasizing the joy of being active in the great outdoors.

I have a loving family, two wonderful boys, now grown up. They have their own lives now and are very happy. Yet still the passion for outdoors is there. In their spare time, our eldest son highlights his adventurous spirit, ignited by the sea's call to explore. Whether it's paddle boarding, or diving into the depths to witness the underwater world, or where the swimming waves take him. The youngest however also has a love for the outdoors. He is someone who is deeply passionate about maintaining and promoting a healthy lifestyle. He values physical activity not just as a means to stay in shape, but as a cornerstone of overall well-being. Encompassing both mental and physical health. Both my husband and I are extremely lucky to have such talented young men.

Dean Forest, Gloucestershire:

This is one of the oldest surviving ancient woodlands in England. It is known for its natural beauty.

We traveled to the Forest of Dean back in June 2017, and stayed at Forest Holidays in a beautiful log cabin at a place called Coleford - Berry Hill, Gloucestershire. One of the many great memories was when we went to a place called Puzzlewood. It is a unique and enchanting site, captivating woodlands. It has been inspired by many artists, writers and filmmakers, including J.K. Rowling.

The forest is noted for its secret caves, ancient trees, and complex of pathways winding dense moss-covered rocks. The site is also family friendly offering treasure hunts and other activities for children, making it a magical outing for visitors of all ages.

Also in the Forest of Dean Gloucestershire, is a place called Symonds Yat which is located along the River Wye with its surrounding forest hills, renowned for its picturesque village. The area is celebrated for its breathtaking views and outdoor activities. Walking, hiking, canoeing, rock climbing, and bird watching are among the most popular pursuits here. The Yat Rock viewpoint, in particular, is a notable spot that offers panoramic views over the Wye Valley. The village itself offers charming accommodation, pubs, and cafes, making it a destination for nature lovers and outdoor enthusiast.

Whilst staying in your adorable log cabins with Forest Holidays, you may want to explore down through the enchanting woods. Every twist and turn hold a promise of discovery, to lose yourself in nature's mysterious woods. Their are many trails and footpaths that lead you to the Wye Valley offering beautiful views of the surrounding countryside. Totally recommend.

I find solace and rejuvenation in nature's embrace. There's something truly invigorating about just breathing in the fresh air and feeling the gentle touch of sunlight on your skin. Weather it's a stroll through the lush green parks, hiking along scenic trails, or simply basking in the tranquility on natural landscape, I cherish every moment that I spend outdoors, Nature offers me a sanctuary where I can unwind, recharge, and reconnect with the beauty and serenity that surrounds us.

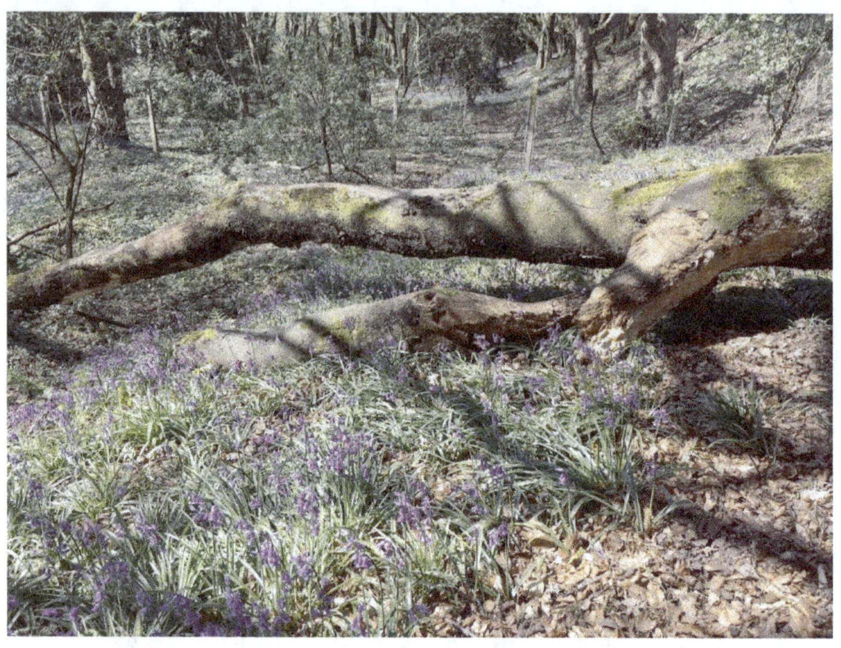

This is my beautiful place known as Bluebell woods in a place called Ringley, Stoneclough, Radcliffe, in Manchester M26 1GT

Introduction to Forest Therapy

Understanding Forest Therapy, also known as forest bathing or Shinrin-yoku in Japanese, is a practice that involves immersing oneself in the natural environment of a forest to enhance health, wellness, and happiness. The concept, which originated in Japan in the 1980's is based on the idea that spending time in nature, particularly forest, can have significant positive effects and mental health. Here's a simplified explanation of its key components.

Connection with Nature

Forest therapy is about reconnecting with nature through our senses. It encourages people to see, smell, taste, touch, and listen to the natural environment around them. This sensory engagement is thought to promote a deeper, more meaningful connection with nature and oneself.

Mindfulness and Relaxation

This practice often involves mindfulness exercises, such as deep breathing, meditation, or guided imagery, which can enhance the therapeutic experiences by promoting and reducing stress. Participants are encouraged to be present in the moment and to release their worries and distractions.

Accessibility

Forest therapy can be practiced in any natural setting, not just in forest. parks, gardens, or even tree-lined streets in urban areas can serve as a suitable environment for forest bathing. The key is to be in a natural environment where one can interact with nature through the senses.

Core Principles of Forest Bathing

Mindfulness and Presence:

The importance of being fully present in the experience, engaging all five senses to connect with the natural environment.

Connection to Nature:

Encouraging a deep, reciprocal relationship with nature, recognizing that humans are part of the natural world and not separate from it.

Healing Through Nature:

Understanding how nature acts as a therapist, offering a space for reflection, healing and rejuvenation.

The Practice of Forest Therapy

Guided walks vs. Solo Experience:

While forest therapy can be done individually, there are also guided sessions where certified forest therapy guides lead participants through a series of invitations to help deepen their connection with the natural world. These guided sessions can provide a structured way to experience forest therapy for beginners.

Typical Activities:

Description of common practices within forest therapy, such as mindful walking, sit spot exercises, meditation practices focused on deepening the connection with nature.

There is no greater way to escape the troubles of daily life, than to find the welcoming embrace of the forest. Here we can breathe more freely and think more clearly our hearts and minds fed with oxygen released by the leaves. Its our special place where we can choose who comes and goes. Its our magical place where we can be fully be who we are, answering our deepest question about ourselves and revealing our most hidden secrets, dreams and desires.

The Essence of Forest Bathing (Shinrin-Yoku)

Introduction

Shinrin-Yoku is built on the premise that nature has a powerful influence on our health. The practice is guided by principles that encourage us to slow down, be present, and engage all our senses. The the core principles of forest bathing including mindfulness, the importance of the natural setting, and the role of sensory engagement in forming a deep connection with nature.

The Science behind the Healing Power of Nature

Scientific research has begun to uncover the mechanisms through which forest bathing exerts its beneficial effects. Studies Suggest that exposure to forest can lower the blood pressure, reduce stress hormone levels, boost immune function, and improve feelings of happiness and creativity. The current scientific understanding of why shinrin-yoku is beneficial, including discussions on phytoncides, natural compounds emitted by trees, and their impact on human health.

phytoncides are natural compounds produced by plants and trees, functioning as a defense mechanism against harmful insects, animals, and microorganisms. These volatile organic compounds are released into the air and can have various beneficial effects on human health when inhaled.

Benefits for Mind, Body, and Soul

The practice of forest bathing offers a multitude of benefits that encompass physical, psychological, and emotional well-being. Participants often report improved mood, reduced anxiety, and a greater sense of focus and clarity. This section has provided a comprehensive overview of the benefits associated with Shinrin-yoku, supported by anecdotal evidence and scientific research.

Distinction Between Forest Therapy and Other Nature Therapies

While forest therapy shares similarities with other nature-based therapies and practices, it also has distinct characteristics that set it apart. This part of the chapter differentiates shinrin-yoku from other approaches, such as wellness therapy, ecotherapy, and garden therapy, highlighting its unique focuses on immersive sensory experiences and the therapeutic use of forest environments.

Conclusion:

Embracing the Essence of Forest Bathing

In embracing the essence of forest bathing, we reconnect with the natural world and rediscover the inherent healing power of nature. The reflections on the importance of integrating shinrin-yoku into our lives, offering guidance on how to begin this enriching practice and incorporate its principles into our daily lives.

By understanding the essence of forest bathing, readers can better appreciate its potential to transform our relationship with nature and ourselves, leading to a more balanced, healthy, and fulfilling lives.

As we prepare to conclude our journey through the forest today, remembering the forest does not rush, yet everything is accomplished in its own time. Carry this sense of peace and the gentle pace of nature with you as you transition back into the bustling world. May the calmness, clarity and connection you've experienced here stay with you guiding your steps and enriching your days. Remember, this forest is always here for you, a sanctuary of peace amidst the chaos of daily life. You're welcome to return in body or spirit whenever you seek tranquility, inspiration, or a sense of belonging. Until next time, let us walk gently on the earth, with respect for all living things.

Preparing for your Forest Therapy Journey

E ngaging with trees in such a picturesque setting can stir emotions of awe and wonder, instilling a peace that calms the mind and rejuvenates the spirit.

In essence, the emotional bond we form with trees in beautiful places is a reflection for our innate longing for connection-not just with nature but with the essence of life itself.

Setting intentions for Your Journey

Before stepping into the forest, it's crucial to set intentions for your forest therapy session. This process involves reflecting on what you hope to achieve or experience, such as seeking peace, clarity or a deeper connection with nature. Knowing how to align your mindset with your intentions, creating a purposeful foundation to your journey.

Selecting the Right Environment

Not all forest and natural settings offer the same experience. The choice of environment be it a dense old grown forest, a tranquil park with scattered trees, or a rugged mountainous area-can significantly influence your forest therapy session. Consider the most suitable environment for your needs, also factors such as accessibility, safety, and the type of nature experience you seek.

Essential Gear and Considerations

While forest therapy encourages simplicity, certain essential items can enhance your experience and ensure safety. From appropriate clothing for varying weather conditions to a water bottle for hydration, this section lists the essentials for a comfortable and safe therapy session. Additional considerations, such as leaving electronics behind to fully immerse in the experience are also discussed.

Clothing

Comfortable, Weather-Appropriate Clothing:

Wear layers that can be easily added or removed based on the temperature. Opt for moisture wicking fabrics to keep you dry.

Waterproof jacket or Raincoat:

In case of unexpected rain it is always good to be prepared.

Long Pants:

To protect your legs from scratches, insect bites, and sun exposure.

Comfortable Walking Shoes:

Waterproof hiking shoes or boots with a good grip are ideal for navigating forest terrain

Hat and Sunglasses:

For protection against the sun and to reduce glare.

Gloves:

Lightweight gloves can be useful in cooler temperatures or to protect your hands

Essentials

Backpack:

To carry your items hands-free.

Water Bottle:

Staying hydrated is crucial, especially if you;ll be walking for long periods of time.

Snacks:

Bring energy-boosting snacks like nuts, fruits or similar energy bars.

Map and Compass/GPS:

If you're in a large or unfamiliar forest, having navigational tools is important.

First Aid Kit:

Always be prepared for minor injuries with band-aids, antiseptic wipes, and any personnel medications.

Insect Repellent:

To protect against ticks, mosquito, and other insects.

Sunscreen:

To protect your skin from UV rays, even in shaded areas.

Camera or Smartphone:

For capturing the beauty of nature (optional, but recommended for those who wish to take memories home).

Notebook and Pen:

Some people find it enriching to jot down thoughts, sketches, or observations.

Binoculars:

Great for bird watching or observing wildlife from a distance.

Mindset and Expectations

Approaching forest therapy with an open mind and unrealistic expectations is the key to embroidering whatever experience nature offers. It explores the importance of letting go of specific outcomes and allowing the natural world to guide your experience. It also addresses common misconceptions and encourages an attitude of curiosity and non-judgment.

Timing and Duration

The optimal timing and duration of a forest therapy session can vary widely depending on individuals preferences and the specific context of the visit. It's advisable to consider and determine the best time of day and length of time to spend in the forest, considering factors like weather, personal energy levels, and the changing seasons.

Solo vs. Guided Sessions

Deciding whether to embark on a forest therapy journey alone or with a guide can affect your experience. There are many benefits and challenges of solo and guided sessions, providing insight into each option catering to different needs and preferences. The choice between solo and guided forest walking depends on what you're looking to get out of the experience. If you value solitude, flexibility and personal reflection. Solo walking might be more suitable. However if you prefer a social, educational experience with the added security of a guide, guided walks would be the better option. Both forms of walking offer significant health benefits and the opportunity to connect with nature.

Safety and Respect for Nature

Safety is paramount when venturing into the forest. It emphasizes the importance of preparing for potential hazards and practicing Leave No Trace principles to minimize your impact on the natural environment. What you require for navigating safety, recognizing and respecting wildlife, and preserving the integrity of natural sites are provided.

By preparing thoughtfully for your forest therapy journey, you can create a meaningful and enriching experience that nurtures your connection with nature and supports your well-being. This chapter equips readers with the knowledge and tools needed to approach forest therapy with confidence, respect, and a sense of wonder.

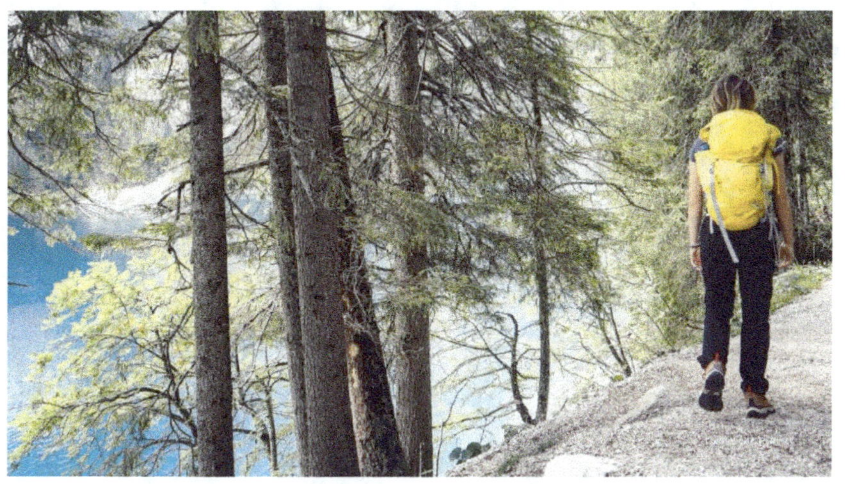

Guided Forest Therapy Techniques

Guided forest therapy techniques aim to deepen participant's connection to nature, enhancing well-being through carefully structured activities that engage the senses, promote mindfulness, and foster a sense of peace and belonging in the natural world. Here are some techniques used in guided forest therapy sessions.

Sensory Awakening

Invitation to Notice:

Guides invite participants to become aware of what is immediately noticeable to their senses. This might involve focusing on the breath, feeling the air on the skin, or listening to the subtle sounds of the forest.

Touch and Texture Exploration:

Participants are encouraged to touch the bark of the trees, feel the texture of leaves, and perhaps walk barefoot to connect directly with the ground.

Mindful Walking

Slow-paced Walks:

Emphasizing slowness to allow for a deeper sensory experience, guides lead participants on gentle walks, encouraging them to notice each step and the sensation of moving through space.

Walking Meditation:

This involves walking in silence, focusing on the movements of the body and the breath, observing nature without judgment.

"With each step I take, I walk in peace, fully present and aligned with the rhythm of the earth."

Deep Listening

Sounds Baths:

Participants sit or lie down in a comfortable spot and close their eyes to focus solely on the sounds around them, allowing the symphony of nature to fill their awareness.

Echo of the Forest:

Guides might encourage participants to vocalize sounds or tones and and listen to the echoes or responses from the environment, fostering a sense of connection and communication.

Visual Immersion

Sit Spot:

Participants choose a spot to sit quietly and observe the environment around them, using the opportunity to notice details they might otherwise overlook.

Visual Scanning:

Guides invite participants to scan the environment at varying speeds and scopes, minutiae of the forest floor to the expansive sky above, encouraging a broad appreciation of nature's diversity.

Olfactory Engagement:

Scent Sharing:

Participants are invited to smell different natural objects, such as leaves, soil or tree bark, and share their experience and memories associated with those scents.

Aromatic Walks:

Walking through areas with rich natural fragrances, participants focus on the smells of the forest, which can have a profound calming effect.

"In the embrace of the woods, my mind is clears, and I connect deeply with the tranquil beauty"

Tasting Nature:

Foraging with Caution:

Under the guidance of an expert, participants may taste edible plants, berries, or herbs found in the forest, connecting with nature through the sense of taste. This is done with utmost caution to ensure safety.

Reflection and Sharing:

Circle of Sharing:

After activities, participants are invited to share their experiences, thoughts, or feelings in a supportive group setting, fostering a sense of community and shared experience.

Nature Art:

Participants might create simple art from natural materials found on the ground, expressing their connection to nature through creativity.

Guided forest therapy sessions are adaptable and can be tailored to the specific group or individual's needs, ensuring that everyone regardless of physical ability or experience with nature can benefit from this immersive healing practice.

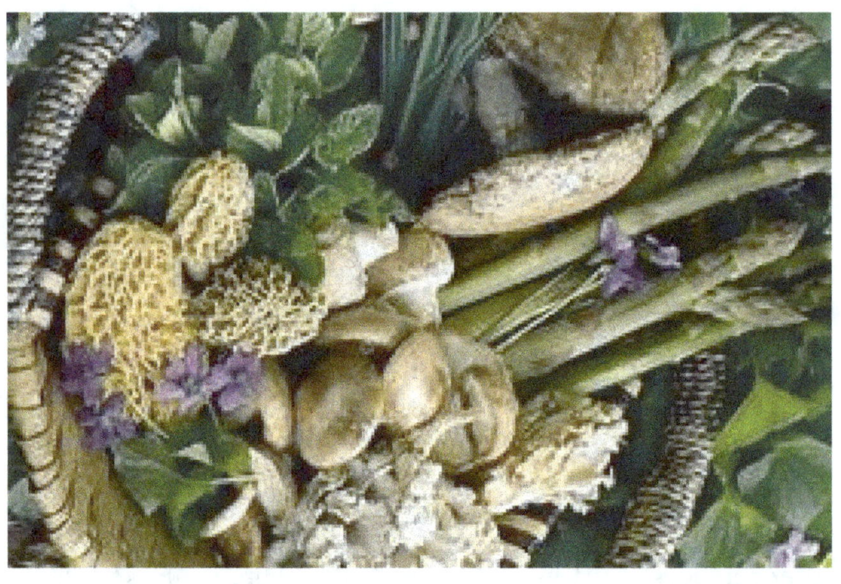

"Natures's Bounty: A quiet pursuit in the Forest's Embrace"

Integrating Forest Therapy into Daily Life

The Importance of Nature in Daily Life

In our fast-paced, technology-driven world, integrating forest therapy into daily life can serve as a vital counterbalance, promoting mental clarity, emotional resilience, and physical well-being. This chapter explores practical ways to weave the principles of forest therapy into the fabric of everyday life, fostering a sustained connection with nature.

Creating a Personal Nature Ritual

Developing a personal nature ritual can anchor your connection to the natural world,even amidst urban environments. Suggestions include:

Morning Moments:

Starting the day with a few minutes of outdoor time, perhaps enjoying a cup of tea or coffee outside to set a calm, grounded tone for the day.

Nature Breaks:

Incorporate short, regular breaks into your day dedicated to connecting with nature. This could mean a brief walk, tending to house plants, or simply standing outside to feel the sun on your face.

Bringing the Outdoors in

Indoor Plants and Micro-Gardens:

Cultivate a collection of indoor plants or create a small herb garden in your kitchen. These green spaces can improve air quality and bring a sense of calm into your home.

Nature Decor:

Use elements from nature to decorate your living and working spaces. Stones, shells, wood, and dried flowers can all serve as reminders of the natural world.

"In the presence of my indoor plants, I find serenity and strength, reminding me of nature's resilient beauty.

Mindful Moments with Nature

Sensory Exercises:

Practice engaging your senses with whatever natural elements are available to you, even in an urban setting, Listen for birds song, smell rain on concrete, or watch for movement of the clouds

Nature Meditation:

Dedicate time for meditation or mindfulness practices that focus on nature-based imagery sounds, such as recording or a forest or ocean.

Incorporating Nature into Work and Leisure

Green Commutes:

Choose routes that pass through parks or along waterways for your daily commute, or if working from home, take walking meetings or breaks in the nearby green spaces.

Nature-Based Hobbies:

Adopt hobbies that encourage time outdoors, such as bird watching, gardening, nature photography, or plane air painting.

Community Engagement and Advocacy

Volunteer for Green Causes:

Engage with your community by volunteering for environmental projects, such as tree planting, community garden maintenance, or local clean-up events.

Promote Green Spaces:

Advocate for the creation and preservation of green spaces within your community, emphasizing the health and wellness benefits they provide.

Seasonal Adaptations

Seasonal Activities:

Tailor your nature interactions to the seasons, embracing the unique aspects of each. This could involve snowshoeing in winter, wildflower walks in spring, swimming in natural bodies of water in summer, hiking to observe autumn foliage.

Indoor Nature Engagement:

During less hospitable seasons, focus on indoor nature engagement, such as building a terrarium, pressing leaves, or crafting with natural materials.

Digital Detoxes and Nature

Scheduled Technology Breaks:

Regularly scheduled time where you disconnect from digital devices to reconnect with your surroundings, promoting mental clarity and stress reduction.

Nature Apps and Tools:

Use technology wisely by leveraging apps that encourage outdoor exploration, such as plant identification apps, trails finders, stargazing guides, to enrich your experiences.

The Ongoing Journey

Integrating forest therapy into daily life is an evolving process, reflecting personal growth and a deep understanding with the natural world. It encourages a lifestyle that values and seeks out the tranquility and rejuvenation found in nature, leading to improved mental, emotional, and physical health.

This chapter aims to inspire readers to find innovative and accessible ways to bring the essence of the forest into their lives, nurturing a continuous and restorative bond with nature.

"Like a tree I stand tall and strong, adapting to each season with grace and courage."

The Healing Power of Trees and Plants

Unveiling Nature's Pharmacy

The natural world offers a vast repository of healing powers, with trees and plants playing a pivotal role in both traditional and modern medicine. This chapter delves into the remarkable abilities of flora to heal, soothe, and enhance human health, highlighting the scientific basis behind the traditional wisdom.

Trees offer a plethora of health benefits related to the concept of "flora," which generally refers to plants in a particular area, but can also hint at the beneficial bacteria (flora) that live in our guts and on our skin. When we talk about health benefits of trees in relation to flora, we're primarily considering the environment and direct physiological benefits they provide, which can indirectly support our body's own flora by promoting a healthy living environment. Here are just a few of the key health benefits.

Air Quality Improvement:

By Improving air quality, trees can indirectly benefit our respiratory health, which is closely linked to our overall immune system and the health of our body's flora.

Mental Health Benefits:

Exposure to green spaces, including areas rich in trees, has been linked to reduced levels of stress, anxiety, and depression. This mental health improvement can support a healthier immune system.

Noise Reduction:

Trees can act as a sound barrier, reducing noise pollution. This can lead to lower stress levels and higher quality of life, indirectly supporting immune and gut health.

Physical Health:

Access to green spaces and tree-dense areas encourages physical activity, whether it's walking, running, or other forms of exercise. Physical health is directly linked to gut health, as regular exercise can improve gut motility and the balance of gut microbiota.

Emotional and Psychological Well-being

Green Therapy:

The psychological benefits of interacting with trees and plants, such as reduced stress, anxiety, and depression. The concept emphasizes the therapeutic effect of being in the forest and natural settings, suggesting that such environments can significantly improve a person's emotional, psychological,and physical health.

Therapeutic Gardens:

The design and use of gardens and green spaces for therapeutic purposes in hospitals, schools and community centers. These gardens are carefully planned to provide a restorative and peaceful environment that can help reduce stress, improve mood, and encourage physical activity.

Spiritual Significance of Trees

Spiritual Growth and Enlightenment:

Trees are often used for spiritual growth and enlightenment. Their steady growth towards the light, while remaining connected to the earth through their roots, can symbolize the human quest for spiritual awakening while staying grounded in physical reality.

Healing Medicinal Properties:

Many cultures believe in the healing powers of trees, using various parts of trees in traditional medicine. Beyond their physical healing properties, trees are also sought for their calming and restorative effects on the human spirit, offering a space for meditation, reflection and connection with the divine.

Personal and Collective Memory:

Trees often serve as living memorials, standing witness to history and connecting generations. They can embody personal memories or represent collective experiences, serving as a silent observer to the passage of time and the stories of a community.

Here's a brief overview of the healing power of plants and trees:

Aromatherapy Properties:

Essential oils extracted from plants are used in aromatherapy to promote physical and psychological well-being. Lavender, for instance, is widely used for its calming and relaxing effects, which can help reduce stress and improve sleep.

Nutritional Benefits:

Plants are essential sources of nutrients, including vitamins, minerals, fiber, and antioxidants, which are crucial for maintaining health and preventing chronic diseases. Fruits, vegetables, nuts, and seeds are integral parts of a healthy diet.

Conservation:
Protecting Nature's Healing Agents

The Importance of Biodiversity:

Discussing the critical role of preserving plant and tree diversity for health of the planet and future medicinal discoveries.

Sustainable Practices:

Encouraging Sustainable interactions with nature, including responsible foraging, supporting conservation efforts, and advocating for the protection of natural habitats.

Conclusion: A Return to the Roots

This chapter concludes by reaffirming the intrinsic connection between human health and the natural world. It calls for a deeper appreciation and respect for trees and plants, not only as sources or physical healing but as essential components of our psychological and spiritual well-being. By fostering a relationship with the natural world, we can unlock the vast potential of nature's pharmacy.

The Future of Forest Therapy

Embracing the woods and nature as our future is a testament to our deep connection with the natural world.

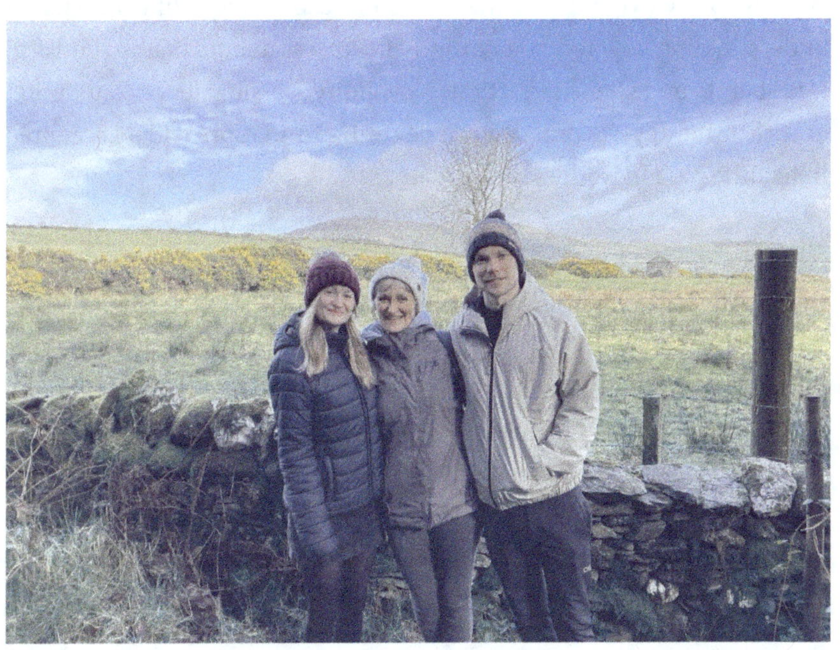

Our favorite pastime, walking in nature through the hills and trees with family. This picture was taken in Archallangan Forest in the Isle of Man, February 2024. Incredibly enlightening to be with family when you're walking. Thank you to all x

Forest therapy has been gaining popularity as a natural way to address the stress and hustle or modern life. Looking into the future, the potential development and integration of forest therapy into mainstream wellness practices could unfold in several promising ways.

Increased Scientific Research:

As interest in forest therapy grows, we can expect more scientific studies to investigate its benefits. This research will likely focus on understanding how forest environments affect mental health, physical well-being, and stress reduction. By solidifying the science foundation of forest therapy, its practice can be refined and more widely accepted in healthcare and wellness industries.

Integration into Healthcare Systems:

Forest therapy might become a prescribed treatment for various conditions, such as anxiety, depression, and stress-related illnesses. Healthcare professionals could recommend forest therapy as part of a holistic treatment plan, potentially in collaboration with parks, nature reserves, and therapeutic professional trained forest in forest therapy.

Expansion of Forest Therapy Trails and Parks:

With growing popularity, we might see the development of more designated forest therapy trails and parks. These areas would be specifically designed to maximize the therapeutic benefits of spending time in nature, with features like guided trails, quiet resting spots, and educational programs about the local ecosystem.

Visual and Augmented Reality Experiences:

For those unable to access natural forest easily, technology could play a role in providing virtual forest therapy experiences. Virtual and augmented reality could stimulate the sensory experiences of being in a forest, making forest therapy accessible to individuals in urban environments or with mobility issues.

Global and Educational Programs:

Businesses and educational institutions may incorporate forest therapy into their wellness and curriculum programs, Recognizing the benefits of reduced stress and improved well-being, these organizations could offer forest therapy sessions as a way to enhance productivity, creativity and overall mental health.

Community and Social Initiatives:

Community-led forest therapy programs could emerge, focusing on social connection, environmental education, and promotion of mental health. These initiatives might work towards making forest therapy accessible to a wider audience, including undeserved communities.

The future of forest therapy looks promising, with potential for significant growth and integration into various aspects of society. As awareness and scientific understanding of its benefits increase, forest therapy could become a cornerstone of natural wellness and mental health strategies.

Community and Belonging

The Green Thumbs Group:

A narrative about a community gardening project that brought people together from diverse backgrounds, creating a sense of belonging and mutual support. The garden became a place of healing for many, including refugees and residents facing social isolation, showcasing the communal healing power of working with plants.

Forest Friends Program:

Highlighting a program that pairs seniors with young volunteers for nature walks, this story emphasizes the cross-generation connections and mutual learning that can happen when people come together in nature. The program not only improved physical health but bridged the gaps of understanding and loneliness.

Solo Group Sessions

In the forest, the heart finds its solace and peace,
A love that's unwavering, that will never cease.
For among the tall trees, where wild spirits roam,
Is a love profound, where all souls find home.

So let us wander, hand in hand, under the green,
In the forest of love, where the world is serene.
With every step, let our hearts more closely knit,
For the embrace of the woods, true love does sit.

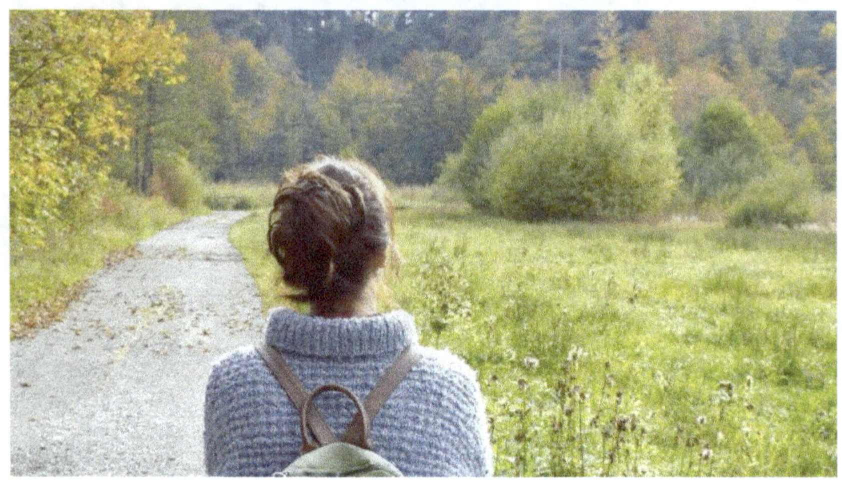

"Being free in nature, I embrace the openness of the outdoors, the vastness of the sky, and the rich tapestry of life that surrounds me. As I breathe in the fresh, crisp air. I am reminded of the boundless possibilities that lie ahead. I am connected beneath my feet, feeling grounded and secure, yet entirely free to explore, to dream, and to be myself without limits. At this moment, I am part of the natural world, sharing in its cycles and its rhythms. I let go of my worries and the constraints of everyday life, finding peace, strength, and renewal a midst the trees, the water, and the wildlife. Hear, in the embrace of nature, I am truly free."

Solo group sessions, often referred to as Shinrin-Yoku or forest bathing, combine the benefits of solo meditation with the group dynamics of guided therapy sessions, albeit in a unique setting. These sessions are designed for individuals within a group to experience the healing powers of nature independently while still benefiting from a structured program that a group setting offers. This experience emphasizes personal reflection and connection with nature, without the pressures of social interaction or the need to engage in group activities.

Participants are guided into a forest or natural setting, where they are encouraged to engage with their surroundings through all their senses. The facilitator might provide prompts or activities designed to deepen the participants connection to the environment, such as mindful walking, deep breathing, identifying natural sound, or gently touching the textures of the leaves and the tree bark. Although the participants are part of a group, each person embarks on their solo journey within the safety and structure the group provides.

The benefits of solo group sessions in forest therapy include reduced stress, improved mood, increased focus, and a deeper sense of connection to the natural world. These sessions can offer a unique way for individuals to tap into their therapeutic aspects of nature, combining the introspection of solo experience with the communal safety and shared intention of group activities.

"Alone in the forest, I find clarity, and a deep sense of peace, reconnecting with myself and the world around me."

Personal Stories of Transformation

I ntroduction

The transformative power of forest therapy is not just a matter of scientific study but is vividly illustrated in the personal stories of those who have experienced its profound impact. This chapter shares a collection of narratives that highlight the diverse and life-changing journeys individuals have embarked on through their engagement within nature.

Healing Beyond Medicine

The Story of Emma:

After a diagnosis of chronic anxiety, Emma found in the forest therapy a sanctuary that medication and traditional therapy had not fully provided. Her regular walks in the local arboretum became a vital part of her healing process, offering her a sense of peace and grounding.

Mark's Recovery:

A veteran struggling with PDSD known as post traumatic stress disorder. Mark's introduction to forest therapy through a rehabilitation program offered him a new lens to view his healing. The tranquility of the forest allowed him to process his trauma, gradually reducing his reliance on medication and improving his relationships.

Re-connection and Discovery

Liam's Journey:

Disenchanted with his high-stress corporate job, Liam turned to forest therapy as a way to disconnect from the pressures of urban life. What began as weekend excursions turned into a life-changing decision to pursue a career in environmental conservation, reconnecting with his childhood love for the outdoors.

Sara's Awakening:

Living in a densely populated city, Sara felt a deep disconnection from nature until a visit to a national park awakened her to the beauty of the natural world. This experience sparked a passion for environmental advocacy, leading her to become an active voice in local green initiatives.

Spiritual and Philosophical Insights

Maya's Transformation:

Maya's experience in forest led her to a deep spiritual awakening, where she found a profound sense of interconnectedness with all living things. Her story illustrates how forest therapy can transcend physical and mental health benefits, touching on spiritual dimensions.

The Philosopher's Path:

A philosopher recounts how regular solitary hikes in the forest have influenced his thinking and writing, providing not only a peaceful retreat but also a source of inspiration and insight into the human condition.

Advocacy and Action

Alex's Mission:

After witnessing the therapeutic effects of forest walks on his own mental health, Ales embarked on a mission to increase urban green spaces. His advocacy has resulted in the development of several community parks and green ways, demonstrating the ripple effect of personal transformation into community action.

The Universal Language of Nature

The stories shared in this chapter underscore the universal appeal and benefits of the forest therapy, transcending cultural age, and socio-economic barriers. They remind us of the essential truth that a our well-being is deeply entwined with the health of the natural world. These personal journeys of transformation through the forest therapy illuminate the path for others, encouraging a collective movement towards embracing nature as a vital component of health and happiness.

"I am healing, growing stronger, and more vibrant everyday. Love and healing energy flow through me renewing my body, mind and spirit"

"With every sunrise, I feel stronger and more at peace, trusting in my body's natural ability to heal and rejuvenate"

The Emerald Isles: A Tapestry of Green

In the annals of natural beauty, the United Kingdom holds a place of honor. A constellation of islands where greenery reigns supreme, it boasts some of the most diverse and enchanting forests in the world. From the misty woodlands of Scotland to the ancient, story-laden groves of England, and the rugged, untamed copse of Wales, these forests are not just a testament to nature's artistry but also a cornerstone of Britain's cultural and ecological heritage.

What makes the United Kingdom truly exceptional is the intricate tapestry of landscapes interwoven across a relatively modest expanse. It's a land where dense, moss-laden forests can be found just a stone's throw from quaint, bustling villages. Where the haunting call of a distant cuckoo echoes through timeless oaks, and where the rustle of leaves underfoot tells tales as old as time. The UK's forests are more than just collections of trees; they are living, breathing remnants of ancient times, serving as guardians of the past and sanctuaries for the present.

Each forest in the UK tells a different story, painted against a backdrop of historical and geographical diversity. In the lush boughs of the Scottish Highlands, one finds solace in the sheer rawness of nature. The dense pine and birch forests, interspersed with heather-clad moorlands and serene lochs, are a tribute to the untamed spirit of the land. These forests, bathed in the soft, golden light of a Highland sunset, are realms of quiet introspection and profound natural beauty.

Journey south, and you enter the verdant heartlands of England. Here, forests like Sherwood in Nottinghamshire and the New Forest in Hampshire are steeped in lore and legend. Sherwood, synonymous with Robin Hood, embodies the adventurous spirit of medieval England. The New Forest, a royal hunting preserve of William the Conqueror, is a mosaic of ancient woodlands and wild heaths, where ponies roam free, unbounded by the tethers of time. These forests are not just a green refuge; they are a bridge to a storied past, echoing with the footfalls of kings and outlaws alike.

Wales, with its rugged landscapes and Celtic heritage, offers a contrasting tapestry of woodlands. The Welsh forests are wilder, more mystical. They are lands where myths and reality intertwine, where every glade could be the dwelling place of an ancient druid or a mythical creature. The forests of Snowdonia, where gnarled oaks stand guard amidst cascading waterfalls and misty peaks, are a testament to Wales' enchanting natural allure.

The beauty of the UK's forests is matched by their ecological significance. These woodlands are vital havens of biodiversity. They are home to a myriad of species, from the elusive badgers and majestic stags to the myriad of bird species that flit through the canopy. Each forest ecosystem plays a crucial role in preserving the environmental health and balance of the region, acting as green lungs and natural sanctuaries.

As one wanders through these forests, it becomes clear that they are more than just spaces of natural beauty; they are chapters in the United Kingdom's story. Each tree, each clearing, each meandering stream has witnessed the passage of time, from ancient history to modern-day. They have been silent spectators to the evolving narrative of a land and its people.

In today's fast-paced world, where concrete jungles often overshadow natural ones, the forests of the UK stand as bastions of tranquility and timeless beauty. They remind us of the need to connect with nature, to find peace amidst the leaves and solace under the boughs. They are not merely places to visit but to experience — to breathe in deeply and emerge rejuvenated, with a newfound appreciation for the natural world.

In conclusion, the forests of the United Kingdom are not just geographical features on a map; they are the heart and soul of the isles. A journey through these green corridors is a journey through history, nature, and oneself. They are the green jewels in the crown of the British Isles, each forest a unique gem with its own hue, story, and song. As we delve into the individual tales of these majestic woodlands, let us remember that they are a part of a larger, grander tapestry — one that is quintessentially, unmistakably British.

Sherwood Forest, Nottinghamshire, England

Enchanting History:

A legendary woodland, Sherwood Forest is steeped in folklore, primarily associated with the legendary Robin Hood. This ancient forest's whispering leaves seem to narrate tales of medieval outlaws.

Majestic Flora:

It's home to a stunning collection of ancient oaks, including the world-renowned Major Oak, possibly over a millennium old, with its colossal hollow trunk and sprawling branches.

Local Treasures:

Nearby, the Sherwood Forest Visitor Centre provides immersive experiences. Mansfield and Newark-on-Trent offer historical and culinary delights.

Stay & Slumber:

From the regal Ye Olde Bell Hotel & Spa to the rustic charm of the Forest Holidays Sherwood Forest cabins, accommodation options are diverse. For camping enthusiasts, Sherwood Pines Campsite offers a true forest immersion.

New Forest, Hampshire, England

Verdant Wilderness:

This forest is a spectacular mix of ancient woodlands and open heaths. Its landscape is dotted with free-roaming horses and deer, creating a fairytale-like atmosphere.

Quaint Villages:

Explore the charming villages of Lyndhurst and Brockenhurst, teeming with history and traditional English charm.

Rest & Relaxation:

The area boasts accommodations such as the elegant Montagu Arms Hotel and the cozy New Forest Lodges. Campers can find solace at Hollands Wood Campsite or Ashurst Campsite, both nestled in natural settings.

Grizedale Forest, Lake District, Cumbria, England

Art in Nature:

Renowned for its outdoor sculpture trail, the forest combines artistic endeavors with natural beauty. Its extensive trails offer panoramic lake and mountain views.

Adventurous Escapes:

The Go Ape adventure park and the Lakes Aquarium are nearby attractions, while the quaint village of Hawkshead is a stone's throw away.

Forest Retreats:

Grizedale Lodge and the nearby Forest Side Hotel offer luxurious stays. For a rustic experience, Low Wray Campsite by Lake Windermere provides an idyllic setting.

The Forest of Dean, Gloucestershire, England

Timeless Woodlands:

A blend of ancient forests and historical sites, it's a sanctuary for wildlife and history enthusiasts. The forest's trails beckon walkers and cyclists alike.

Historical Highlights:

Explore the Clearwell Caves and the Dean Forest Railway. The Wye Valley, known for its breathtaking scenery, is also nearby.

Woodland Accommodations:

The historic Speech House Hotel offers a royal stay, while Bracelands Campsite and Forest Holidays' cabins provide more nature-focused lodging options.

Galloway Forest Park, Dumfries and Galloway, Scotland

Starry Nights:

As a Dark Sky Park, it's a paradise for stargazers. The park is a tapestry of dense woodlands, serene lochs, and abundant wildlife.

Nearby Discoveries:

The Scottish Dark Sky Observatory and the quaint town of Newton Stewart are nearby gems.

Lakeside Lodgings:

The Kirroughtree House Hotel and the Galloway Astronomy Centre offer unique stays. Glentrool Camping and Caravan Site presents a delightful camping experience in the heart of nature.

Kielder Forest, Northumberland, England

Astronomical Wonders:

Famous for its observatory and expansive landscapes, Kielder is a haven for nature and astronomy lovers. Kielder Water adds a watersports dimension.

Forest Attractions:

The Kielder Observatory and Kielder Water & Forest Park are must-visits.

Serene Stays:

The Kielder Waterside Lodges offer luxury amidst nature, while Leaplish Waterside Park provides camping opportunities with stunning views.

Epping Forest, London/Essex border, England

Urban Oasis:

This sprawling ancient woodland provides a much-needed green escape for city dwellers. It's a treasure trove of history and nature.

Cultural Expeditions:

Queen Elizabeth's Hunting Lodge and the Epping Forest District Museum are significant landmarks. The town of Loughton offers additional urban comforts.

Diverse Dwellings:

The Waltham Abbey Marriott Hotel and Packfords Hotel offer urban comfort, while Debden House presents a camping experience within the forest bounds.

Snowdonia National Park, North Wales

Mountainous Majesty:

Renowned for its towering peaks, Snowdonia's forests add an enchanting dimension to the rugged landscape, offering serene trails and diverse flora and fauna.

Welsh Wonders:

The challenge of climbing Mount Snowdon, or the exploration of picturesque towns like Betws-y-Coed and Llanberis, make for unforgettable experiences.

Luxurious Lodgings:

Stay at the iconic Hotel Portmeirion or the comfortable Gwesty Seren Hotel. For those seeking a camping experience, Gwern Gôf Isaf Farm offers a picturesque setting perfect for hikers and nature lovers.

Cairngorms National Park, Scottish Highlands

Highland Havens:

The park is home to majestic landscapes, including the ancient Caledonian Pine Forest, offering sanctuary to a diverse range of wildlife and breathtaking natural beauty.

Unique Experiences:

The Cairngorms Reindeer Centre and the scenic Cairngorm Mountain Railway provide unique attractions. The area is also a haven for winter sports enthusiasts.

Highland Retreats:

The opulent Fonab Castle Hotel and the homely Cairngorm Hotel offer luxurious stays. For a closer-to-nature experience, the Rothiemurchus Camp and Caravan Park are set in stunning natural surroundings.

Forest of Bowland, Lancashire, England

Natural Beauty:

An Area of Outstanding Natural Beauty, it's celebrated for its sweeping moorland, tranquil wooded valleys, and vibrant birdlife. It offers a tranquil escape into nature's embrace.

Local Charms:

The Bowland Wild Boar Park and the historic Clitheroe Castle are local attractions not to be missed.

Charming Stays:

The Inn at Whitewell provides luxury in a picturesque setting, while the Bowland Fell Park offers rustic charm. Beacon Fell View Holiday Park is ideal for those wishing to camp amidst natural beauty.

Thetford Forest, Norfolk and Suffolk, England

Expansive Greenery:

As the UK's largest lowland pine forest, Thetford Forest offers a vast landscape of pines, heathland, and broadleaves. It's a paradise for birdwatchers and nature enthusiasts.

Adventure and History:

The forest is rich in history, with ancient sites like Grime's Graves prehistoric flint mines. For adventure, High Lodge offers activities like Go Ape, cycling, and walking trails.

Accommodations:

Choose from forest lodges like the Thorpe Forest or nearby B&Bs in Thetford town. Camping is available at The Dower House Touring Park, offering a serene woodland setting.

Ashdown Forest, East Sussex, England

Literary Landscapes:

Known as the setting for A.A. Milne's Winnie the Pooh stories, Ashdown Forest's heathland and woodlands are steeped in charm and nostalgia.

Walking and Wildlife:

The forest provides extensive walking paths and is a habitat for diverse wildlife, including deer and many bird species.

Stay Nearby:

Accommodations range from the luxurious Ashdown Park Hotel & Country Club to cozy cottages in surrounding villages. For camping, the Blackberry Wood Campsite offers a unique experience among the trees.

Dean Forest, Monmouthshire and Gloucestershire, England and Wales

Cross-border Charm:

Stretching across England and Wales, this forest is rich in varied landscapes, with wooded gorges and industrial heritage sites.

Local Exploration:

Visit the enchanting Puzzlewood, an ancient woodland that inspired J.R.R. Tolkien. The Dean Forest Railway offers scenic rides through the forest.

Accommodation Choices:

Stay in charming cottages or at the Bells Hotel and the Speech House Hotel. For camping, the Whitemead Forest Park provides excellent facilities in a picturesque setting.

Hatfield Forest, Essex, England

Ancient Woodlands:

One of the oldest hunting forests in England, Hatfield Forest is a remarkable example of a medieval royal hunting park with its ancient trees and deer herds.

Nature Activities:

Ideal for walking, cycling, and bird watching, the forest also offers picturesque lake views perfect for picnics.

Local Stays:

Nearby hotels like The White House offer comfortable accommodation. For a more adventurous stay, camping is available within the forest grounds.

Dalby Forest, North Yorkshire, England

Activity Hub:

This forest in the North York Moors National Park is known for its extensive network of walking and cycling trails, and it's also a popular venue for concerts and events.

Star Gazing:

Dalby Forest is part of the North York Moors Dark Sky Reserve, making it an excellent location for stargazing.

Diverse Accommodation:

Stay at the nearby Dalby Forest Lodges or opt for camping at the Dalby Forest Campsite to truly immerse yourself in the natural environment.

Argyll Forest Park, Argyll and Bute, Scotland

Scottish Splendor:

Part of the Loch Lomond and The Trossachs National Park, this forest park offers stunning landscapes of mountains, lochs, and woodlands.

Outdoor Adventures:

It's a haven for hikers, cyclists, and wildlife enthusiasts. The park also offers water sports on Loch Long and Loch Eck.

Accommodations:

The area boasts a range of options, from luxury lodges like the Ardgartan Argyll Lodges to quaint cottages and campsites amidst the lush scenery.

Each of these forests, with their unique charms and offerings, stands as a testament to the UK's rich natural heritage. They provide not just a retreat for those seeking solace in nature, but also a journey into the heart of England's, Scotland's, and Wales' verdant landscapes. Whether it's the legendary allure of Sherwood Forest, the celestial wonders of Galloway Forest Park, or the rugged beauty of the Cairngorms, each forest invites visitors to explore and connect with the natural world in a profound and memorable way.

In these forests, every path leads not just through rows of towering trees and across babbling brooks, but also to discoveries about the land's history, the local culture, and, most importantly, about oneself. The forests of the UK are not merely places; they are experiences waiting to be lived.

Positive Affirmations

P ositive affirmations about life, nature and trees can instill a sense of peace, appreciation, connectedness to the world around us. Here are some affirmations that might help.

"This fresh air is healing me."

"I am renewed by time spent outside."

"I am one with nature and it is one with me."

"I belong here."

"I can feel my spirit being recharged by this sacred time outdoors."

"The richness of nature surrounds me."

"With my feet touching earth, I am grounded and supported."

"The sun on my face warms me and gives me strength."

"I am filled with wonder by nature's designs."

"I am in awe, standing before creation."

"The sounds of nature fill my heart and bring me peace."

"Today, I connect with all the beings around me."

"Nature is nurturing me, helping me flourish."

"I am one with the wind, the trees and the sky."

Conclusion

I n conclusion, forest therapy serves as a compelling reminder of nature's profound impact on our health and happiness. By embracing the serenity and inherent the wisdom of the natural world, we can cultivate a more balanced, healthy, fulfilled life. As we move forward, let us carry with us the lessons learned from the forest of stillness, resilience, and the simple joy of being alive amidst the beauty of the earth.

By immersing ourselves into the tranquility of the forest, we tap into the rich tapestry of benefits for both our physical and mental states. Embracing nature's healing embrace we discover that our well-being is intricately intertwined with the health of the environment.

In this part of the woods, where the trees are so tall they seem to touch the sky, there's a sense of being a small part of something vast and timeless. The majesty of the forest surrounds you, a reminder of the natural world's power and beauty, and the magic that lies in the heart of the woods.

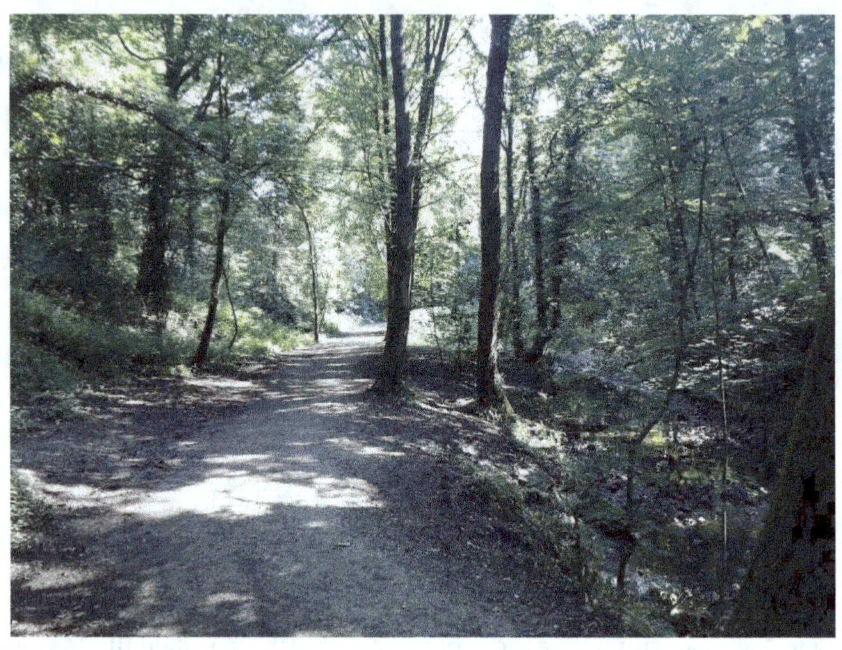

Resources

Wagner, K. D. (2022, April 8). *15 Nature affirmations to embrace the great Outdoors*. Spirituality+Health. https://www.spirtualityhealth.com/articles/2016/04/29/15-affirmations-embrace-great-outdoors

Forest Holidays UK | Cabins & Lodge Holidays. (n.d.). https://www.forestholidays.co.uk/

www.ingramcontent.com/pod-product-compliance
Lightning Source LLC
Chambersburg PA
CBHW071550260726
48653CB00007BA/2621